Chapter 1: Introduction to Eczema

What is Eczema?

Eczema, also known as atopic dermatitis, is a chronic skin condition characterized by inflamed, itchy, and often painful patches of skin. It can vary in severity and can appear in different forms, but its hallmark symptoms include dryness, redness, and itchiness. While eczema can affect individuals of all ages, it is particularly common in infants and children, with many experiencing their first symptoms within the first year of life. Understanding eczema is crucial for patients as it helps in recognizing triggers and managing symptoms effectively.

The causes of eczema are multifactorial and involve a combination of genetic, environmental, and immunological factors. Individuals with eczema often have a compromised skin barrier, which makes their skin more susceptible to irritants, allergens, and infections. This vulnerability can lead to flare-ups, where symptoms worsen and require more intensive management. Identifying personal triggers—such as certain fabrics, soaps, or environmental factors—can be a key aspect of managing eczema and preventing exacerbations.

Dietary influences can also play a significant role in eczema management. Some patients find that certain foods trigger their symptoms, leading to the consideration of elimination diets or food allergy testing. Common culprits include dairy, eggs, nuts, and gluten. However, it is essential for patients to approach dietary changes carefully, ideally under the guidance of a healthcare professional, to ensure they maintain a balanced diet while identifying potential triggers.

Natural remedies have gained popularity among patients seeking alternative or complementary approaches to managing eczema. Options such as coconut oil, colloidal oatmeal, and probiotics may offer relief for some individuals. While these remedies can be effective for mild cases, it is important to note that they may not work for everyone, and a comprehensive skincare routine that includes moisturizing and proper cleansing is critical in managing the condition. Always consult with a healthcare provider before trying new treatments.

The impact of eczema extends beyond the physical symptoms, affecting mental health and quality of life. Many individuals with eczema report feelings of embarrassment, frustration, and anxiety related to their appearance and the unpredictability of flare-ups. This emotional burden can be particularly pronounced in children and adolescents, making it essential for caregivers to provide support and understanding. Awareness of the psychological aspects of living with eczema can enhance overall management strategies, leading to a more holistic approach to treatment and care.

Types of Eczema

Eczema, also known as atopic dermatitis, is a common chronic skin condition characterized by inflammation, redness, and itching. There are several types of eczema, each with distinct symptoms and triggers, which can complicate diagnosis and treatment. Understanding these types is crucial for patients seeking effective management strategies. The most prevalent forms include atopic dermatitis, contact dermatitis, dyshidrotic eczema, nummular eczema, and seborrheic dermatitis. Each type can affect individuals differently based on age, skin type, and environmental factors.

Atopic dermatitis is the most common type of eczema, frequently seen in infants and children but can persist into adulthood. It often presents as dry, itchy patches, typically found on the face, scalp, and inside the elbows and knees. Patients with atopic dermatitis may also experience flare-ups triggered by allergens, irritants, or stress. This type of eczema is associated with other allergic conditions, such as asthma and hay fever, indicating a potential genetic predisposition. Understanding this association can help in managing symptoms effectively through a comprehensive approach that includes skincare routines and dietary considerations.

Contact dermatitis occurs when the skin reacts to a specific substance, such as soaps, detergents, or metals. It is divided into two categories: irritant contact dermatitis, resulting from direct skin irritation, and allergic contact dermatitis, which occurs when the immune system reacts to an allergen. This type of eczema is more common in adults and can lead to localized rashes that can be itchy and inflamed. Identifying and avoiding triggers is essential for effective management, and patients often benefit from keeping a detailed record of their exposures to pinpoint potential irritants or allergens.

Dyshidrotic eczema is characterized by small, itchy blisters that typically appear on the hands and feet. This type can be particularly frustrating for patients, as the blisters can become painful and may lead to cracking or peeling of the skin. Stress and seasonal changes, especially during warm weather, are common triggers for dyshidrotic eczema. Management strategies may include topical treatments, oral medications, and lifestyle adjustments that focus on reducing stress and maintaining skin hydration.

Nummular eczema, often mistaken for ringworm, presents as coin-shaped patches of irritated skin that can be extremely itchy. This type of eczema typically occurs after the skin has been dry or damaged, and it can affect any part of the body. Moisturizing frequently and using topical steroids can help alleviate symptoms. Lastly, seborrheic dermatitis commonly affects areas rich in oil glands, such as the scalp and face, leading to greasy, scaly patches. This form is often linked to yeast overgrowth and may require antifungal treatments. Understanding these various types of eczema enables patients to better recognize their symptoms and seek appropriate treatment, ensuring a more effective management plan tailored to their specific needs.

Common Symptoms

Eczema is a chronic skin condition that manifests through a range of symptoms, which can vary widely from person to person.

Understanding these common symptoms is essential for effective management and treatment. The most recognizable symptom of eczema is dry, itchy skin. This itchiness can often lead to scratching, which exacerbates the condition by causing further irritation and inflammation. In infants and children, this symptom may present as restless behavior or difficulty sleeping, while adults may experience a more persistent itch that can significantly affect their quality of life.

In addition to itchiness, eczema is characterized by redness and inflammation of the affected areas. The skin may appear swollen and warm, indicating an inflammatory response. This redness often occurs in patches, which can be localized or more widespread depending on the severity of the eczema. In infants, the most common areas for eczema flare-ups include the cheeks and scalp, while older children and adults may notice symptoms on the hands, elbows, or behind the knees. Recognizing these patterns can help in identifying triggers and implementing preventative measures.

Another common symptom of eczema is the formation of scaly or flaky skin. This occurs when the skin's barrier function is compromised, leading to moisture loss and subsequent dryness. In some cases, eczema can also result in thickened skin, known as lichenification, which develops from chronic scratching and irritation. This thickening can make the skin appear leathery and can contribute to the discomfort associated with eczema. Maintaining a regular skincare routine that focuses on hydration can help alleviate these symptoms and prevent further skin damage.

Eczema can also lead to oozing and crusting in more severe cases. This is often a result of secondary infections that occur when the skin's protective barrier is compromised. These infections can exacerbate symptoms and lead to increased redness, swelling, and discomfort. It is crucial for patients, especially parents of infants and children, to monitor for signs of infection, such as increased pain, warmth, or pus, and seek medical advice when necessary. Effective management strategies, including topical treatments and hygiene practices, can help reduce the risk of complications.

Lastly, the emotional and psychological impact of eczema should not be underestimated. Many patients experience anxiety, frustration, or low self-esteem as a result of their condition. This is particularly evident in children who may face bullying or social exclusion due to their visible symptoms. Adults may also find their professional and personal lives affected by the self-consciousness stemming from their skin condition. By acknowledging the mental health aspects of eczema, patients can seek appropriate support and incorporate holistic approaches, such as mindfulness and stress management techniques, into their overall treatment plan. Understanding and addressing both the physical and emotional symptoms of eczema is vital for achieving a better quality of life.

Chapter 2: Eczema in Infants and Children

Recognizing Eczema in Young Children

Recognizing eczema in young children is essential for early intervention and effective management. Eczema, also known as atopic dermatitis, often presents as red, dry, itchy patches on the skin. In infants and toddlers, the condition commonly affects areas such as the face, scalp, and the creases of the elbows and knees. It is crucial for parents and caregivers to familiarize themselves with these signs, as early recognition can help prevent the condition from worsening and can lead to a more effective treatment plan.

The appearance of eczema can vary significantly among children. In younger infants, the rash may appear as small, red bumps that can ooze and crust over, while older children might develop thicker, scaly patches that can become more pronounced with scratching. Understanding these variations is important, as they can lead to different approaches in managing the symptoms. Additionally, eczema can exacerbate during certain seasons, particularly in dry or cold weather, making it vital for caregivers to monitor their child's skin condition during these times.

Dietary influences can also play a significant role in the severity and frequency of eczema flare-ups in children. Some children may have food allergies or sensitivities that contribute to their eczema symptoms. Common allergens include dairy, eggs, peanuts, and gluten. Keeping a food diary can help identify potential triggers, allowing parents to consult with healthcare professionals regarding dietary adjustments or allergy testing. By recognizing the link between diet and eczema, caregivers can take proactive steps to minimize flare-ups.

In managing eczema, natural remedies can be beneficial alongside conventional treatments. Moisturizers and emollients are crucial for

maintaining skin hydration, especially after bathing. Products that contain natural ingredients such as oatmeal or coconut oil might soothe irritated skin and provide relief from itching. It is important, however, to consult with a healthcare provider before introducing any new treatments, as individual reactions can vary. Establishing a consistent skincare routine that includes gentle cleansing and moisturizing can create a protective barrier for sensitive skin.

Lastly, the psychological impact of eczema on young children should not be overlooked. The visible nature of eczema and associated itching can lead to feelings of self-consciousness, frustration, and anxiety. Parents and caregivers should be attentive to their child's emotional needs and be proactive in discussing their condition in a positive light. Encouraging children to express their feelings and providing support can help mitigate the mental health challenges associated with living with eczema. By recognizing the condition and its broader implications, caregivers can foster a supportive environment that promotes both physical and emotional well-being.

Treatment Options for Infants

Treatment options for infants with eczema require a careful and gentle approach, as their skin is particularly sensitive and still developing. The primary goal of treatment is to alleviate symptoms, reduce inflammation, and prevent flare-ups. Moisturization plays a crucial role in this process. Infants benefit from regular application of emollients, which help to lock in moisture and create a protective barrier on the skin. It is advisable to use fragrance-free and hypoallergenic products specifically formulated for infants, as these are less likely to irritate their delicate skin.

When it comes to topical treatments, mild corticosteroids are commonly prescribed for managing inflammation during flare-ups. These medications can effectively reduce itching and redness when used as directed. For infants, physicians typically recommend low-potency corticosteroids for short periods to minimize potential side effects. In some cases, more advanced treatments such as calcineurin inhibitors may be considered. These non-steroidal options can help manage eczema without the same risks associated with steroid use and are suitable for sensitive areas like the face and genitals.

Dietary influences can also play a significant role in managing eczema in infants. Parents should consult with a pediatrician or a dermatologist to evaluate potential food allergies or sensitivities that might exacerbate the condition. Common allergens such as dairy, eggs, and nuts may need to be eliminated from the infant's diet, particularly if there is a family history of atopic diseases. In breastfeeding mothers, dietary adjustments may also be beneficial, as allergens can be transmitted through breast milk. Keeping a food diary can help identify triggers and facilitate discussions with healthcare providers.

Natural remedies are often sought by parents looking for gentle alternatives to conventional treatments. Some options include oatmeal baths, which can soothe irritated skin and provide moisture, and natural oils like coconut oil or sunflower oil that can enhance skin hydration. However, it is essential to approach these remedies cautiously and consult with a healthcare professional before introducing them, as some natural products can also cause irritation or allergic reactions in sensitive infants.

Finally, managing eczema in infants requires an understanding of the emotional impact on both the child and the parents. Eczema can lead to discomfort and disrupted sleep, which can affect the overall well-being of the infant and create stress for caregivers. It is crucial for parents to seek support and share their experiences with others who understand the challenges of managing eczema. Regular check-ups with healthcare providers can also help ensure that treatment plans are effective and adjusted as necessary, providing both the infant and the family with the best possible quality of life.

Long-term Management

Long-term management of eczema requires a comprehensive approach that encompasses various strategies tailored to individual needs. For patients, especially parents managing eczema in infants and children, it is crucial to establish a consistent skincare routine. This routine should include regular moisturization to maintain skin hydration and barrier function. Emollients should be applied frequently, ideally after bathing or whenever the skin feels dry. In addition to maintaining skin moisture, patients should carefully monitor for any products that may exacerbate symptoms, opting for fragrance-free and gentle formulations.

Dietary influences play a significant role in the management of eczema. Patients should be aware of potential food triggers that can lead to flare-ups. Common allergens such as dairy, eggs, nuts, and wheat may exacerbate symptoms for some individuals, particularly in children. Keeping a food diary can help identify correlations between dietary intake and eczema flare-ups. Consultation with a healthcare professional or a dietitian can assist in determining an appropriate elimination diet and ensuring nutritional needs are met, especially when managing eczema in young children.

Natural remedies are often sought by patients looking for alternatives or complementary therapies to conventional treatments. Ingredients like colloidal oatmeal, coconut oil, and honey have shown promise in soothing irritated skin and reducing inflammation. However, it is essential to approach natural remedies with caution, as not all products are suitable for every individual. Patch testing new products on a small area of skin can help prevent adverse reactions. Ensuring these remedies are part of a broader management plan that includes medical advice is vital for achieving the best outcomes.

Mental health should not be overlooked in the long-term management of eczema. The chronic nature of the condition can lead to feelings of frustration, anxiety, and depression, impacting quality of life. Patients should seek support from mental health professionals if they experience significant emotional distress related to their eczema. Additionally, joining support groups or connecting with others who share similar experiences can provide valuable emotional support. A holistic approach that addresses both physical symptoms and mental health can lead to better overall management of the condition.

Finally, understanding and managing triggers is essential for long-term eczema care. Seasonal changes can significantly impact symptoms, with dry winter air or pollen in spring exacerbating conditions for many individuals. Identifying personal triggers, such as stress, heat, or certain fabrics, is crucial for developing effective avoidance strategies. Regular follow-ups with a healthcare provider can help patients adapt their management plans as needed, ensuring that both flare-ups and the emotional toll of living with eczema are effectively managed.

Chapter 3: Dietary Influences on Eczema

Foods That May Trigger Eczema

Foods that may trigger eczema can vary significantly from person to person, making it essential for patients to identify their individual sensitivities. Common culprits often include dairy products, eggs, nuts, soy, wheat, and shellfish. These foods contain proteins that can provoke an immune response in some individuals, leading to inflammation and exacerbation of eczema symptoms. It is crucial for patients to observe their reactions to different foods and consider keeping a food diary to track any correlations between their diet and skin flare-ups.

In infants and children, the introduction of new foods can coincide with the onset of eczema. Parents should be particularly cautious when introducing common allergens. Research suggests that early exposure to certain allergens may either increase the risk of developing eczema or help in building tolerance. For example, introducing small amounts of peanut products at an early age has been shown to reduce the likelihood of developing peanut allergies. However, it is vital to consult with a healthcare provider before making any significant changes to a child's diet, especially if they have a family history of allergies.

Adults with eczema may also find that specific foods exacerbate their symptoms. Beyond the common allergens, some individuals report that processed foods high in sugar and unhealthy fats can trigger flare-ups. These foods can lead to systemic inflammation, which may worsen eczema. Incorporating a diet rich in whole foods, such as fruits, vegetables, whole grains, and healthy fats, can help manage and potentially reduce eczema symptoms. Patients should aim for a balanced diet that supports overall skin health and immune function.

Natural remedies often complement dietary changes in managing eczema. Many patients explore options such as probiotics, which may help balance gut bacteria and improve skin health. Omega-3 fatty acids, found in fatty fish and flaxseed, are also known for their anti-inflammatory properties and may assist in reducing eczema symptoms. Patients should discuss any natural remedies with their healthcare provider to ensure they align with their overall treatment plan and do not interfere with prescribed medications.

Lastly, understanding the link between diet and mental health is essential for patients with eczema. Flare-ups can lead to emotional distress, which may create a cycle of worsening symptoms. A balanced diet not only supports physical health but also contributes to improved mood and well-being. Patients may benefit from consulting with a dietitian or nutritionist who specializes in eczema to tailor a dietary plan that addresses both their physical symptoms and emotional health, ultimately leading to a more holistic approach to managing eczema.

Anti-inflammatory Diets

Anti-inflammatory diets have gained attention in recent years as a promising approach to managing various health conditions, including eczema. These diets focus on reducing systemic inflammation through the consumption of specific foods while minimizing the intake of inflammatory agents. For patients dealing with eczema, understanding how dietary choices can impact inflammation is crucial in managing symptoms and improving overall skin health. This subchapter will explore the principles of anti-inflammatory diets, their potential benefits, and practical tips for incorporating these dietary strategies into daily life.

At the core of an anti-inflammatory diet is the emphasis on whole, nutrient-dense foods. Patients are encouraged to consume a variety of fruits, vegetables, whole grains, lean proteins, and healthy fats. Foods rich in omega-3 fatty acids, such as fatty fish, walnuts, and flaxseeds, are particularly beneficial as they possess anti-inflammatory properties. Additionally, incorporating colorful fruits and vegetables can provide essential vitamins, minerals, and antioxidants that help combat oxidative stress, which is often linked to skin inflammation and eczema flare-ups.

Certain foods should be limited or avoided in an anti-inflammatory diet to help manage eczema symptoms. Processed foods, refined sugars, and trans fats can exacerbate inflammation and trigger allergic reactions in some individuals. Dairy products and gluten may also be problematic for certain patients, especially those with sensitivities. Keeping a food diary can be a valuable tool for identifying personal triggers and understanding how specific foods influence eczema symptoms on an individual basis.

In addition to food choices, the timing of meals and overall lifestyle habits can play a significant role in inflammation levels. Consuming regular, balanced meals can help stabilize blood sugar levels and prevent spikes in inflammation. Staying hydrated is also crucial, as water aids in skin hydration and helps flush out toxins. Moreover, integrating other anti-inflammatory practices, such as regular physical activity, stress management techniques, and adequate sleep, can further enhance the effectiveness of dietary changes in managing eczema.

While adopting an anti-inflammatory diet can be beneficial for many patients, it is important to approach dietary changes thoughtfully and in consultation with healthcare professionals. Each individual's experience with eczema is unique, and what works for one person may not be suitable for another. Collaborating with a registered dietitian or nutritionist can help patients develop a personalized plan that considers their specific needs, preferences, and possible food sensitivities. By integrating an anti-inflammatory diet into their overall eczema management strategy, patients may find relief from symptoms and improve their quality of life.

Keeping a Food Diary

Keeping a food diary can be a valuable tool for individuals managing eczema, as it allows for a systematic approach to identifying potential dietary triggers that may exacerbate symptoms. This practice involves recording everything consumed on a daily basis, including meals, snacks, beverages, and any additional supplements. By meticulously noting food intake, patients can gain insights into how their diet may correlate with flare-ups or changes in their skin condition. This detailed record can serve as a foundational element in discussions with healthcare providers, enabling a more tailored approach to treatment and management.

When maintaining a food diary, it is essential to include not just the foods consumed, but also the time of consumption and any accompanying symptoms experienced afterward. Patients should note the severity of their eczema symptoms, skin reactions, and any other relevant observations such as stress levels, sleep quality, or environmental factors. This comprehensive approach can help establish patterns and connections that might otherwise be overlooked. For instance, a patient may discover that dairy products lead to increased itchiness or that certain fruits trigger rashes, thus providing critical information for dietary adjustments.

In the case of infants and children with eczema, keeping a food diary can be particularly beneficial for parents aiming to identify potential allergens or irritants in their child's diet. Young children are often more susceptible to certain foods, and their reactions may differ from those of adults. By monitoring dietary intake and skin responses, parents can work closely with pediatricians or dietitians to eliminate specific foods from their child's diet. This can lead to improved skin health and overall well-being, reducing the frequency and severity of eczema flare-ups.

It is important to approach the food diary with consistency and honesty, recording all items without omission. This can be challenging, especially in busy households or when dining out, but the benefits can be significant. Patients may consider utilizing smartphone applications or online platforms designed for food tracking, which can simplify the process and make it easier to analyze data over time. Additionally, sharing this information with healthcare providers can facilitate a more effective evaluation of dietary influences on eczema, leading to informed recommendations and possible dietary modifications.

In conclusion, keeping a food diary is an empowering practice for those managing eczema, providing clarity and direction in the pursuit of symptom relief. By recognizing the relationship between diet and skin health, patients can take proactive steps to minimize flare-ups and enhance their quality of life. Whether for adults, children, or infants, this method serves as an essential tool in developing a comprehensive management plan that addresses both immediate symptoms and long-term skin health.

Chapter 4: Natural Remedies for Eczema

Herbal Treatments

Herbal treatments have gained popularity as complementary options for managing eczema symptoms. Many individuals seeking alternatives to conventional medications are turning to natural remedies derived from plants. These treatments can provide relief from itching, inflammation, and dryness, making them appealing for patients of all ages, including infants and children. However, it is crucial to approach herbal remedies with caution, as not all products are created equal, and some may even exacerbate symptoms.

Common herbal treatments for eczema include chamomile, calendula, and aloe vera. Chamomile, known for its anti-inflammatory properties, can soothe irritated skin and reduce redness. Calendula is often used in creams and ointments to promote healing and provide moisture to dry skin. Aloe vera is widely recognized for its cooling effect and ability to hydrate the skin, making it a popular choice for those dealing with flare-ups. When considering these remedies, patients should opt for high-quality products and consult with healthcare professionals to ensure safety and efficacy.

The dietary influences on eczema cannot be overlooked when exploring herbal treatments. Certain herbs, such as turmeric and ginger, possess anti-inflammatory properties that may help reduce eczema flare-ups when incorporated into a balanced diet. Additionally, some patients report improvements when avoiding known allergens or irritants, such as dairy or gluten. Including herbs that support gut health, like peppermint and fennel, may also play a role in managing eczema symptoms, as a healthy gut can influence overall skin health.

It is essential for patients to understand the importance of patch testing before fully integrating any herbal treatment into their skincare routine. This step helps to identify potential allergic reactions or irritations that may arise from specific herbs. Applying a small amount of the herbal product to a discreet area of the skin can provide insights into how the skin will react. Alongside this, maintaining a consistent skincare regimen that includes moisturizing and gentle cleansing can enhance the effectiveness of herbal remedies.

While herbal treatments can be beneficial, they should not replace conventional medical advice or treatments. Patients should maintain open communication with their healthcare providers to ensure a holistic approach to managing eczema. By combining the insights gained from herbal treatments with traditional methods, individuals can develop a comprehensive plan tailored to their specific needs. This integrative approach can improve overall quality of life and help patients navigate the challenges associated with eczema more effectively.

Essential Oils

Essential oils have gained considerable attention in recent years as a natural remedy for various skin conditions, including eczema. These concentrated plant extracts are known for their therapeutic properties, which may help alleviate some symptoms associated with eczema, such as dryness, irritation, and inflammation. When considering essential oils as part of an eczema management plan, it is crucial to understand their potential benefits, how to use them safely, and which oils are most effective for this condition.

Among the many essential oils available, lavender oil is often highlighted for its calming and soothing effects. Studies suggest that lavender oil can help reduce inflammation and promote healing, making it a popular choice for those suffering from eczema. Additionally, tea tree oil, recognized for its antimicrobial properties, may help prevent infections that can complicate eczema flare-ups. When diluted appropriately with a carrier oil, these essential oils can be incorporated into skincare routines, offering a natural alternative to commercial products that may contain harsh chemicals.

Safety is a primary concern when using essential oils, especially for infants and children with eczema. Essential oils should always be diluted before application to avoid skin irritation or allergic reactions. A patch test is advisable to determine how the skin reacts to a specific oil. If you're considering using essential oils for a child, consult with a pediatrician or dermatologist to ensure appropriate usage and to choose oils that are safe for their age group. Infants and young children may have more sensitive skin, so caution is essential.

Dietary influences on eczema also play a role in how essential oils can be utilized in managing symptoms. Certain essential oils, such as chamomile and peppermint, can be ingested in small amounts to help reduce inflammation from within. However, it is vital to approach this method with care and to consult a healthcare professional before incorporating any oils into your diet. Understanding the connection between diet and eczema can enhance the effectiveness of essential oils as part of a holistic treatment strategy.

In addition to their physical benefits, essential oils can also positively impact mental health, which is particularly important for individuals dealing with the emotional toll of eczema. The aroma of certain oils, like bergamot and frankincense, can promote relaxation and alleviate stress, potentially reducing the frequency and severity of eczema flare-ups triggered by anxiety. Integrating essential oils into daily routines, whether through topical application or aromatherapy, may not only help manage physical symptoms but also support emotional well-being, offering a more comprehensive approach to eczema care.

Lifestyle Changes

Lifestyle changes play a crucial role in managing eczema symptoms effectively. For patients dealing with eczema, especially infants and children, understanding the impact of daily routines and environmental factors can significantly influence their skin health. Simple adjustments in lifestyle can lead to improved skin conditions, reducing flare-ups and enhancing overall well-being. Patients are encouraged to adopt a proactive approach in identifying their triggers and modifying their environments accordingly.

Dietary influences on eczema have gained increasing attention in recent years. Certain foods may exacerbate symptoms, while others can help soothe inflamed skin. Patients should consider keeping a food diary to track their diet and any corresponding changes in their eczema. Introducing anti-inflammatory foods, such as fatty fish, leafy greens, and nuts, may provide relief. Conversely, common allergens like dairy, nuts, or gluten should be monitored, particularly in children whose immune systems are still developing. Consulting with a healthcare provider or nutritionist can help tailor a diet that supports skin health.

In addition to dietary considerations, exploring natural remedies can complement traditional treatments. Many patients have found relief through the use of natural oils, such as coconut oil and jojoba oil, known for their moisturizing properties. Herbal remedies, such as chamomile and calendula, can also soothe irritated skin. However, it is essential to patch-test any new products to avoid adverse reactions. Embracing a holistic approach by incorporating natural remedies into a daily skincare routine can enhance the management of eczema symptoms.

Mental health is another critical aspect of managing eczema, as the condition can take a toll on emotional well-being. Patients often experience anxiety, frustration, or embarrassment due to their symptoms, which can lead to a cycle of stress and worsening eczema. Practicing stress-reduction techniques, such as mindfulness, yoga, or deep breathing exercises, can be beneficial. Support groups or counseling may also provide a safe space for patients to share their experiences and coping strategies, promoting a healthier mental state.

Lastly, understanding seasonal changes and their effects on eczema can help patients prepare and adapt their routines accordingly. Cold, dry air in winter can lead to increased skin dryness, while summer heat may trigger sweating and irritation. Adjusting skincare regimens to include more intensive moisturizers during dry months and lightweight, breathable fabrics in warmer weather can help maintain skin hydration. By being proactive and responsive to these changes, patients can better manage their eczema and improve their quality of life.

Chapter 5: Eczema and Mental Health

The Emotional Impact of Eczema

The emotional impact of eczema extends far beyond the physical symptoms of the condition. Patients often experience feelings of frustration, embarrassment, and isolation due to the visible nature of eczema. For many, the constant itching and discomfort can lead to significant distress, affecting their overall quality of life. Children with eczema may struggle with self-esteem issues, especially when they notice differences between their skin and that of their peers, which can lead to social withdrawal or bullying. Understanding these emotional ramifications is crucial for both patients and caregivers in addressing the complete well-being of those affected by eczema.

In infants and children, the emotional toll of eczema can manifest in various ways. Parents often feel helpless when they see their child in discomfort, leading to heightened anxiety and stress. Additionally, the relentless nature of flare-ups can disrupt daily routines, including sleep patterns, which in turn affects the entire family. For children, the inability to explain their discomfort can lead to frustration and tantrums, as they do not fully understand why they feel the way they do. Creating a supportive environment that acknowledges these feelings can help families cope better with the emotional challenges posed by eczema.

Dietary influences can also play a significant role in the emotional experience of eczema. Many patients report that certain foods exacerbate their symptoms, leading to a cycle of anxiety around eating. This can create a sense of isolation, particularly for children who may feel different during social occasions involving food. It is essential for patients to work closely with healthcare providers to identify dietary triggers and develop an eating plan that minimizes flare-ups while fostering a positive relationship with food. This proactive approach can alleviate some of the emotional burden associated with managing eczema.

Natural remedies for eczema may offer additional emotional support for patients. Many individuals seek alternative treatments to help manage their symptoms, which can lead to a sense of empowerment and control over their condition. Engaging in holistic approaches, such as mindfulness, yoga, or herbal remedies, can provide emotional relief and help reduce stress, which is known to be a trigger for eczema flare-ups. Establishing a personalized skincare routine that incorporates natural products may also promote a sense of comfort and security, helping patients feel better physically and emotionally.

Lastly, the intersection of eczema and mental health cannot be overlooked. Studies suggest that individuals with eczema are at a higher risk of developing anxiety and depression. The visible nature of the condition can lead to feelings of shame and inadequacy, impacting social interactions and personal relationships. It is vital for patients to seek support, whether through counseling, support groups, or educational resources, to address the emotional aspects of living with eczema. Open discussions about mental health and eczema can reduce stigma, foster understanding, and ultimately improve the emotional well-being of those affected.

Coping Strategies

Coping strategies play a vital role in managing eczema effectively, providing patients with practical methods to alleviate symptoms and improve their quality of life. Understanding the triggers specific to each individual is the first step in creating a personalized approach. Keeping a symptom diary can be particularly useful; by documenting flare-ups alongside dietary choices, skincare routines, and environmental factors, patients can identify patterns that may contribute to their eczema. This awareness empowers patients to make informed decisions about their lifestyle and treatment options.

For infants and children, coping strategies often involve creating a supportive environment that minimizes irritation. Parents should focus on dressing their children in breathable, soft fabrics, and avoiding harsh detergents and irritants. Establishing a consistent skincare routine is crucial; regular moisturizing with appropriate emollients can help maintain skin barrier function and prevent dryness. Additionally, engaging children in their care can help them understand their condition better, promoting a sense of control and reducing anxiety related to flare-ups.

Dietary influences on eczema are significant, and patients should consider incorporating anti-inflammatory foods into their diets. Foods rich in omega-3 fatty acids, such as fatty fish, flaxseeds, and walnuts, may help reduce inflammation, while probiotics found in yogurt can support gut health. Conversely, common allergens such as dairy, nuts, and gluten may exacerbate symptoms for some individuals. Consulting with a nutritionist can provide tailored dietary advice, helping patients to navigate their food choices without feeling deprived.

Natural remedies can also serve as effective coping strategies for managing eczema symptoms. Ingredients like coconut oil, aloe vera, and oatmeal baths are known for their soothing properties. However, it's essential to approach natural remedies with caution, as some individuals may have sensitivities to certain substances. Patients should conduct patch tests and consult with their healthcare providers before introducing new treatments to ensure they do not exacerbate their condition.

Mental health is an often-overlooked aspect of coping with eczema. The visible nature of the condition can lead to feelings of embarrassment, frustration, and isolation. It is crucial for patients to seek support from mental health professionals, support groups, or online communities where they can share experiences and coping strategies. Engaging in stress-reducing activities such as yoga, meditation, or mindfulness practices can further enhance emotional well-being. By addressing both the physical and emotional aspects of eczema, patients can develop a holistic approach to managing their symptoms and improving their overall quality of life.

Seeking Professional Help

Seeking professional help is a crucial step for anyone struggling with eczema, whether it is a mild case or a more severe form affecting daily life. Consulting a healthcare professional, such as a dermatologist, can provide you with a proper diagnosis and a tailored treatment plan. Dermatologists specialize in skin conditions and are well-equipped to identify the specific type of eczema you may have, along with its underlying causes. This expertise is particularly beneficial for patients dealing with eczema in infants and children, as treatment approaches may differ significantly from those used for adults.

In addition to dermatologists, other healthcare professionals such as allergists and nutritionists can play a vital role in managing eczema. Allergists can help identify potential allergens that may trigger flare-ups, while nutritionists can guide dietary changes that may alleviate symptoms. For many patients, understanding the links between diet and eczema can lead to significant improvements in their condition. For instance, eliminating certain foods known to trigger eczema symptoms can reduce flare-ups and improve overall skin health.

The emotional and psychological impact of eczema cannot be understated, especially in children and adults who experience visible symptoms. Seeking professional help can also include mental health support, as individuals with eczema may struggle with anxiety, depression, or low self-esteem due to their condition. Therapists who specialize in chronic illnesses can provide coping strategies and emotional support, helping patients manage the mental health aspects of living with eczema. This holistic approach to treatment recognizes that managing eczema isn't just about skin care but also about emotional well-being.

When it comes to skincare routines, professionals can offer guidance on the most effective products and practices tailored to individual skin types and sensitivities. A dermatologist can recommend specific emollients, moisturizers, and topical medications that may help control symptoms and prevent flare-ups. Moreover, they can advise on safe and effective natural remedies, ensuring they do not interfere with prescribed treatments. Establishing a consistent skincare routine under professional guidance can lead to better management of symptoms and an overall improvement in skin condition.

Lastly, follow-up appointments with healthcare providers are essential for monitoring progress and adjusting treatment plans as needed. Eczema can change over time due to seasonal variations, lifestyle changes, or new exposures. Regular consultations allow for timely interventions and adaptations to your management plan, ensuring you remain equipped to handle your eczema effectively. Whether you are experiencing eczema for the first time or have been living with it for years, seeking professional help is a proactive step towards achieving better skin health and a higher quality of life.

Chapter 6: Eczema in Adults

Adult Eczema Symptoms

Adult eczema, also known as atopic dermatitis, can manifest in various ways, presenting unique symptoms that may differ from those experienced by infants and children. Common symptoms include persistent itching, which can range from mild to severe, causing significant discomfort and sometimes leading to sleep disturbances. The itching often intensifies during dry seasons or in response to irritants, making it critical for patients to recognize their individual triggers and manage them effectively.

In adults, the skin affected by eczema may appear red, inflamed, and dry. Lesions can develop on various parts of the body, including the hands, elbows, and behind the knees. These patches can become crusty or scaly, and in some cases, they may ooze or bleed if scratched excessively. The appearance of the skin can lead to feelings of self-consciousness, affecting one's mental health and social interactions. Recognizing these physical symptoms is vital for developing a comprehensive management plan.

Another significant symptom of adult eczema is the tendency for skin to become thickened or leathery over time, a condition known as lichenification. This occurs due to chronic scratching and can contribute to a cycle of itch and irritation, making the symptoms more challenging to manage. Additionally, adult eczema can lead to secondary infections, as the compromised skin barrier is more susceptible to bacteria and viruses. Patients should be vigilant about any signs of infection, such as increased redness, warmth, or pus.

Emotional and psychological symptoms accompanying adult eczema should not be overlooked. Many adults with eczema experience anxiety, depression, or low self-esteem linked to their skin condition. The visible nature of eczema can result in social withdrawal or avoidance of certain situations, further exacerbating mental health challenges. It is essential for patients to address these emotional aspects, potentially seeking support from mental health professionals or support groups.

Effective management of adult eczema symptoms often involves a combination of topical treatments, lifestyle modifications, and possibly dietary adjustments. Patients are encouraged to establish a consistent skincare routine that includes moisturizing frequently and using gentle, fragrance-free products. Identifying and avoiding specific triggers, such as allergens or irritants, can significantly reduce flare-ups. By adopting a holistic approach that considers both physical and emotional well-being, patients can better manage their eczema and improve their quality of life.

Workplace Challenges

Workplace challenges can significantly impact individuals managing eczema, as the environment often exacerbates symptoms. For many, the workplace is a source of stress, which can trigger flare-ups. Factors such as temperature fluctuations, exposure to irritants, and the pressure of meeting deadlines can heighten discomfort. Understanding how these elements interact with eczema is crucial for patients looking to manage their condition effectively.

Exposure to various allergens and irritants in the workplace is a common concern for those with eczema. Many workplaces utilize cleaning products, air fresheners, and office supplies that may contain harsh chemicals. For patients, these substances can lead to skin irritation and worsen existing symptoms. It is essential for individuals to identify potential triggers in their work environment and communicate with employers about necessary accommodations, such as switching to hypoallergenic products or improving ventilation.

Temperature and humidity control are also vital in managing eczema symptoms at work. Offices can often be overly air-conditioned or heated, leading to dry air that can exacerbate skin issues. Patients should consider using a humidifier or keeping moisturizers handy to maintain skin hydration throughout the day. Dressing in layers can help regulate body temperature and reduce discomfort caused by sweating or chills. These small adjustments can create a more conducive environment for managing eczema.

Mental health challenges associated with eczema can further complicate workplace dynamics. Individuals may experience anxiety or embarrassment due to visible symptoms, which can affect their confidence and productivity. It is important for patients to seek support, whether through counseling, support groups, or engaging with colleagues who understand their condition. Developing coping strategies and fostering open communication about eczema can help alleviate some of the mental burden associated with the condition.

Finally, creating a personalized skincare routine that fits seamlessly into a workday is essential for managing eczema effectively. Patients should consider applying moisturizers throughout the day, selecting non-irritating products, and maintaining a consistent routine that aligns with their work schedule. Educating coworkers about eczema can also promote understanding and support, fostering a more inclusive work environment. By addressing these workplace challenges proactively, individuals can better manage their eczema and maintain their overall well-being.

Treatment Options for Adults

Treatment options for adults with eczema are diverse and tailored to individual needs, considering the severity of the condition, the specific symptoms experienced, and any coexisting health issues. Topical therapies remain a cornerstone of eczema management. These include corticosteroids, which reduce inflammation and alleviate itching. Non-steroidal topical agents, such as calcineurin inhibitors, offer an alternative for sensitive areas, minimizing the potential for side effects associated with long-term steroid use. It is crucial for patients to follow their healthcare provider's instructions regarding the strength and frequency of application to ensure efficacy and safety.

Systemic treatments may be appropriate for adults with moderate to severe eczema. These include oral medications like corticosteroids and immunosuppressants, which work by suppressing the immune response that contributes to inflammation. Recent advancements have introduced biologic therapies, specifically designed to target specific pathways in the immune system. These medications can provide significant relief for individuals who have not responded adequately to traditional therapies. However, they require careful monitoring for potential side effects and are usually considered when other treatments have failed.

In addition to pharmacologic treatments, patients should consider integrating lifestyle modifications that can significantly impact their eczema management. Identifying and avoiding triggers is essential; common triggers include stress, allergens, and irritants such as soaps and detergents. Keeping a symptom diary can help patients recognize patterns and make informed choices about their environment and activities. Moreover, maintaining a consistent skincare routine is vital. Gentle, fragrance-free cleansers and moisturizers should be applied regularly to keep the skin hydrated and reduce flare-ups.

Dietary influences on eczema are also a critical area for consideration. Some patients find that certain foods exacerbate their symptoms. An elimination diet, guided by a healthcare professional, may help identify specific dietary triggers. Incorporating anti-inflammatory foods, such as omega-3 fatty acids found in fish and walnuts, can support overall skin health. Staying well-hydrated and avoiding excessive alcohol and caffeine can also contribute to skin wellness. It is advisable for patients to consult with a registered dietitian to develop a balanced diet that supports their skin and overall health.

Lastly, addressing the mental health aspect of living with eczema is essential for comprehensive care. The chronic nature of the condition can lead to anxiety, depression, and social withdrawal. Patients should not hesitate to seek support from mental health professionals or support groups, as sharing experiences can provide comfort and coping strategies. Mindfulness and stress-reduction techniques, such as yoga and meditation, may also prove beneficial. By taking a holistic approach that combines medical treatment, lifestyle modifications, and mental health support, adults with eczema can effectively manage their symptoms and improve their quality of life.

Chapter 7: Eczema Skincare Routines

Daily Skincare Practices

Daily skincare practices play a crucial role in managing eczema symptoms and maintaining skin health. For patients dealing with eczema, establishing a consistent skincare routine can significantly reduce flare-ups and improve overall comfort. The core of this routine involves gentle cleansing, moisturizing, and protection from irritants. Each step should be tailored to individual skin needs, especially in vulnerable populations such as infants, children, and adults who may have varying sensitivities.

Cleansing is the first step in any effective skincare routine. Patients should opt for mild, fragrance-free cleansers that do not strip the skin of its natural oils. It is advisable to avoid hot water, which can exacerbate dryness and irritation. Instead, lukewarm water is recommended for washing affected areas. For infants and children, sponge baths with gentle cleansers can help minimize discomfort while ensuring cleanliness. Patients should also limit the frequency of baths or showers to prevent excessive drying of the skin.

Moisturizing is the cornerstone of eczema management and should be performed immediately after cleansing. A thick, emollient cream or ointment is preferred over lotions, as these products provide a stronger barrier against moisture loss. Applying moisturizer while the skin is still damp can enhance absorption and effectiveness. For infants, using products specifically formulated for sensitive skin can ensure safety and efficacy. Adults may benefit from experimenting with different formulations, including those with added ingredients like ceramides or hyaluronic acid to boost hydration.

Protection from environmental triggers is an essential aspect of daily skincare practices. Patients should identify and avoid known irritants, such as harsh soaps, detergents, and certain fabrics. Wearing soft, breathable clothing can help minimize friction and irritation. Additionally, during seasonal changes or in dry climates, adjusting the skincare routine to include more frequent moisturizing can help combat increased dryness. Using a humidifier at home can also assist in maintaining optimal skin moisture levels, particularly during winter months.

Lastly, patients should be mindful of their mental health, as eczema can have a significant psychological impact. Establishing a calming skincare routine can not only provide physical relief but also serve as a moment of self-care. Incorporating mindfulness techniques, such as deep breathing while applying products, can help reduce anxiety related to flare-ups. Sharing experiences with support groups or healthcare professionals can also provide emotional support and practical advice, ultimately helping patients navigate their eczema management journey with greater confidence and understanding.

Choosing the Right Products

Choosing the right products for managing eczema is crucial for effectively controlling symptoms and improving overall skin health. When selecting skincare products, patients should prioritize those that are specifically formulated for sensitive skin. Look for items labeled as hypoallergenic, fragrance-free, and free from harsh chemicals. These products are less likely to irritate the skin or trigger an eczema flare-up. Reading ingredient lists is essential; avoid potential allergens and irritants such as alcohol, synthetic fragrances, and certain preservatives, which can exacerbate symptoms.

For infants and children, it is particularly important to choose products that cater to their delicate skin. Pediatric dermatologists often recommend emollients and moisturizers that provide a barrier to prevent moisture loss. Creams and ointments are typically more effective than lotions for sealing in hydration. Products containing ceramides, glycerin, and hyaluronic acid can help restore the skin's natural barrier, reducing the likelihood of dryness and irritation. Parents should also test new products on a small area of skin before applying them more broadly.

Dietary influences can play a significant role in eczema management, and patients should consider products that support their nutritional needs. Certain foods may exacerbate symptoms, while others could help soothe the skin. Incorporating foods rich in omega-3 fatty acids, antioxidants, and vitamins A and E can be beneficial. Patients may also explore dietary supplements or natural remedies, but it is essential to consult with healthcare providers to ensure that these options are safe and effective.

When it comes to eczema skincare routines, consistency is key. Patients should establish a daily regimen that includes gentle cleansing followed by generous application of moisturizers. Products that contain colloidal oatmeal or aloe vera can provide additional relief from itching and inflammation. Additionally, incorporating products with anti-inflammatory properties, such as those containing chamomile or calendula, can help soothe irritated skin. Adapting the skincare routine to seasonal changes is also vital, as colder months may require richer creams, while warmer months might call for lighter formulations.

Lastly, understanding the connection between eczema and mental health can guide product choices that promote a sense of well-being. Stress and anxiety can worsen eczema symptoms, so selecting products that offer a sensory experience may be beneficial. Aromatherapy oils or soothing lotions can create a calming atmosphere during application, reinforcing self-care practices. Additionally, patients should seek support from healthcare professionals to address the psychological aspects of living with eczema, ensuring a holistic approach that includes both physical and emotional aspects of care.

Moisturizing Techniques

Moisturizing is a cornerstone of eczema management, as it helps restore the skin's barrier function and prevent moisture loss. For individuals with eczema, the skin often lacks the ability to retain moisture, leading to dryness, irritation, and flare-ups. Selecting the right moisturizer is crucial. Look for products that are free from fragrances, dyes, and common allergens, as these can exacerbate symptoms. Creams and ointments are generally more effective than lotions because they offer a thicker barrier to seal in moisture. Opt for products labeled as hypoallergenic or designed specifically for sensitive skin to minimize the risk of irritation.

When applying moisturizer, timing is essential. The best practice is to apply it immediately after bathing, while the skin is still damp. This technique helps to lock in moisture and enhance the effectiveness of the product. Use a gentle, non-irritating cleanser during baths to avoid stripping the skin of its natural oils, and limit bath time to prevent excessive drying. After patting the skin dry with a soft towel, apply the moisturizer generously over all affected areas. For infants and children, ensure that the moisturizer is applied with care, focusing on areas prone to eczema such as elbows, knees, and the face.

Incorporating a consistent moisturizing routine is beneficial for both children and adults with eczema. Establishing a daily regimen that includes applying moisturizer at least twice a day can significantly improve skin hydration and reduce flare-ups. For infants, caregivers should be diligent about applying moisturizer after diaper changes and baths. For adults, maintaining a portable moisturizer can help manage symptoms throughout the day, especially in response to environmental triggers such as dry air or cold temperatures. Consistency and routine are key elements in managing eczema effectively.

Natural remedies can also play a role in enhancing the moisturizing effects of traditional products. Ingredients such as coconut oil, shea butter, and aloe vera are often well-tolerated and provide additional hydration. When using natural remedies, it is important to conduct a patch test to ensure no allergic reactions occur. Additionally, some patients may find relief with oils such as sunflower or jojoba, which can support the skin barrier. However, these should complement a primary moisturizing routine rather than replace it, as they may not provide sufficient hydration on their own.

Finally, it is essential to recognize the impact of environmental factors on skin hydration. Seasonal changes can influence moisture levels in the air, making it necessary to adjust moisturizing techniques accordingly. During colder months, for instance, indoor heating can lead to dry air, exacerbating eczema symptoms. In such cases, using a humidifier can help maintain moisture in living spaces. Additionally, staying hydrated by drinking plenty of water and following a balanced diet rich in omega-3 fatty acids may support skin health from the inside out. By employing effective moisturizing techniques, patients can take proactive steps in managing their eczema and improving their overall skin health.

Chapter 8: Eczema Triggers and Management

Common Environmental Triggers

Common environmental triggers play a significant role in the exacerbation of eczema symptoms. Understanding these triggers is crucial for patients seeking effective management strategies. Environmental factors can vary widely, including allergens, irritants, and climate conditions that affect the skin's barrier function. Patients often find that specific elements in their daily surroundings can lead to flare-ups, making it essential to identify and minimize exposure to these triggers.

One prevalent environmental trigger is dust mites, microscopic organisms that thrive in household dust. They are particularly troublesome for individuals with eczema, as their droppings can provoke allergic reactions and skin irritation. Regular cleaning, using allergen-proof covers for bedding, and maintaining low humidity levels in the home can help reduce dust mite populations. Patients should also consider washing bedding and soft toys frequently in hot water to eliminate these allergens, providing a more conducive environment for skin health.

Another common trigger is pet dander. For those who are sensitive to animals, dander can cause significant irritation and lead to eczema flare-ups. While it may not be feasible for every family to eliminate pets, strategies such as keeping pets out of bedrooms, using air purifiers, and regularly grooming pets can help minimize exposure. Patients should evaluate their individual reactions to pets and make informed decisions about their living arrangements to reduce the risk of exacerbating their eczema.

Climate and seasonal changes can also impact eczema symptoms. For example, cold weather often leads to dry air, which can strip moisture from the skin and worsen eczema. Conversely, hot and humid conditions can lead to sweating, which can irritate the skin and trigger flare-ups. Patients should adjust their skincare routines according to the season, using thicker moisturizers in the winter and lightweight, breathable fabrics in the summer. Staying hydrated and using humidifiers during dry months can also help maintain skin moisture levels.

Lastly, exposure to various irritants in everyday products can aggravate eczema. Common irritants include soaps, detergents, fragrances, and certain fabrics. Patients should opt for fragrance-free, hypoallergenic products and avoid harsh cleaning agents. Conducting patch tests when introducing new products can help identify potential irritants before they lead to a flare-up. By becoming aware of these common environmental triggers and making necessary lifestyle adjustments, patients can significantly improve their eczema management and overall quality of life.

Stress and Eczema

Stress can significantly impact the severity and frequency of eczema flare-ups. For many patients, the relationship between stress and eczema is complex, as stress can act as both a trigger for flare-ups and a response to the discomfort caused by the condition. When a person experiences stress, the body releases hormones like cortisol, which can lead to inflammation and exacerbate existing skin conditions. Understanding this connection is essential for patients seeking to manage their eczema effectively.

In infants and children, the effects of stress on eczema can manifest differently. Young children may not have the verbal skills to express their feelings, making it challenging for parents to identify stress as a contributing factor to their eczema. Situations such as changes in routine, family dynamics, or environmental stressors can lead to increased discomfort. Parents should be attentive to these potential stressors and address them proactively, as reducing stress can help minimize flare-ups and improve overall skin health.

Dietary influences also play a role in managing stress and eczema. Certain foods may trigger inflammation or allergic reactions, which can further stress the skin. A balanced diet rich in omega-3 fatty acids, antioxidants, and anti-inflammatory foods can help reduce both stress and eczema symptoms. Patients should consider keeping a food diary to identify any correlations between their diet, stress levels, and skin condition. This approach allows for a more personalized management plan that addresses both dietary and emotional triggers.

Natural remedies can offer additional support in managing stress-related eczema. Practices such as mindfulness, yoga, and meditation can help patients decrease stress levels, leading to a potential reduction in flare-ups. Topical natural remedies, including moisturizing agents like coconut oil or shea butter, can soothe irritated skin while also providing a calming effect on the mind. Incorporating these practices into a daily routine can foster resilience against stress, ultimately benefiting both mental health and skin condition.

Maintaining an effective skincare routine is crucial for patients dealing with stress and eczema. Regularly moisturizing the skin helps create a barrier that protects against irritants and allergens that may exacerbate symptoms. Additionally, patients should be encouraged to identify and avoid known triggers, whether they are environmental, dietary, or emotional in nature. By combining stress management techniques with a robust skincare regimen, patients can take control of their eczema and improve their quality of life.

Developing a Management Plan

Developing a management plan for eczema is essential for effectively controlling symptoms and improving quality of life. The first step in creating a personalized management plan involves assessing the severity of the eczema and identifying specific triggers. Patients should keep a detailed diary to track flare-ups, noting any potential environmental, dietary, or emotional factors that may contribute to their condition. This record can help both the patient and healthcare provider understand patterns in symptoms, enabling more targeted strategies for prevention and management.

Once triggers are identified, the next phase is to establish a comprehensive skincare routine tailored to individual needs. This includes selecting suitable moisturizers and topical treatments that hydrate the skin and reduce inflammation. For infants and children, it is crucial to use products that are hypoallergenic and free from harmful chemicals. Adults may also benefit from specialized formulations that address their unique skin concerns. Establishing a consistent routine can help maintain skin barrier function and minimize the frequency and severity of flare-ups.

Dietary influences on eczema cannot be overlooked in a management plan. Many patients find that certain foods exacerbate their symptoms, while others may help to alleviate them. It is advisable for patients to consider an elimination diet under the guidance of a healthcare professional to identify any food allergies or sensitivities. Incorporating anti-inflammatory foods rich in omega-3 fatty acids, antioxidants, and vitamins can also support overall skin health. Patients should discuss their dietary habits with a nutritionist to create a balanced meal plan that complements their eczema management.

Natural remedies can play a significant role in managing eczema symptoms as well. Many patients explore holistic approaches, such as herbal treatments, essential oils, and probiotics. These remedies may provide soothing effects and reduce inflammation. However, it is essential to consult with a healthcare provider before integrating any new treatment into the management plan, as some natural products can cause allergic reactions or interact with conventional medications.

Lastly, it is important to address the mental health aspect of living with eczema, as the condition can significantly impact emotional well-being. Developing coping strategies, such as stress management techniques and seeking support from mental health professionals, can be beneficial. Patients should also consider joining support groups where they can share experiences and advice with others dealing with similar challenges. By combining effective skincare routines, dietary considerations, natural remedies, and mental health support, patients can create a robust management plan that enhances their ability to live comfortably with eczema.

Chapter 9: Eczema and Seasonal Changes

Eczema in Winter

Eczema, particularly atopic dermatitis, can be significantly affected by seasonal changes, with winter presenting unique challenges for those who suffer from this condition. During winter months, the combination of cold temperatures and low humidity levels can lead to drier skin, exacerbating symptoms like itching, redness, and inflammation. Patients often notice that their eczema flares up during this time, making it crucial to understand the seasonal influences on their skin health and to adopt appropriate management strategies.

The dry winter air strips moisture from the skin, diminishing its natural barrier function. For infants and children, whose skin is often more sensitive, this can result in severe itching and discomfort, leading to increased scratching and potential skin infections. Parents should monitor their children's skin closely during winter months and be proactive in maintaining hydration. This may include regular application of moisturizers and emollients that are specifically designed to lock in moisture and create a protective barrier over the skin.

Dietary influences can also play a role in managing eczema in winter. Certain foods may trigger flare-ups, and the winter diet often includes an increase in processed foods and allergens that can aggravate symptoms. Patients should consider keeping a food diary to identify any correlations between their diet and eczema flare-ups. Incorporating anti-inflammatory foods, such as fatty fish rich in omega-3 fatty acids, fruits, and vegetables, may help to improve skin health and reduce the severity of symptoms during the colder months.

Natural remedies can offer additional relief for eczema sufferers during winter. Many patients find that bathing practices need adjustment; taking shorter, lukewarm baths with gentle, fragrance-free cleansers can help prevent further drying of the skin. Following baths, applying thick moisturizers or oils while the skin is still damp can significantly enhance hydration. Additionally, using a humidifier in the home can help to maintain moisture levels in the air, reducing the overall dryness that leads to irritation.

Finally, it's important for patients to be aware of the mental health aspects associated with winter eczema flares. The discomfort and visible signs of eczema can lead to feelings of self-consciousness and frustration, especially in social situations. Engaging in stress-reducing activities such as mindfulness, yoga, or gentle exercise can be beneficial. Seeking support from healthcare providers or support groups may also provide patients with effective coping strategies to manage both the physical and emotional challenges of eczema during the winter months.

Eczema in Summer

Eczema, also known as atopic dermatitis, can present unique challenges during the summer months. The warmer weather and increased humidity often lead to a change in how the condition manifests, with symptoms sometimes becoming more pronounced. Patients may notice that their skin becomes itchier or more inflamed as they spend more time outdoors, exposed to various environmental triggers. Understanding these seasonal fluctuations is crucial for managing eczema effectively.

In summer, sweat can be a significant trigger for eczema flare-ups. As temperatures rise, the body naturally produces more sweat to cool down. For individuals with eczema, this sweat can irritate the skin and exacerbate existing symptoms. It is essential for patients to adopt strategies to manage sweat, such as wearing loose-fitting, breathable clothing and opting for lightweight fabrics that wick moisture away from the skin. Regular bathing to remove sweat and allergens can also help mitigate irritation.

Sun exposure can have both positive and negative effects on eczema. While moderate sun exposure can lead to improvements in some patients' skin conditions, overexposure can result in sunburn, which can further irritate eczema-prone skin. It is essential for patients to find a balance, using sunscreen that is appropriate for sensitive skin and reapplying it regularly. Additionally, protective clothing and seeking shade during peak sun hours can help prevent flare-ups related to sun exposure.

Dietary influences also play a role in managing eczema during the summer. Seasonal foods, such as fresh fruits and vegetables, can contribute to overall skin health. However, patients should remain mindful of potential allergens that may be more prevalent in summer diets, such as certain fruits or nuts. Keeping a food diary can assist in identifying any dietary triggers that correlate with flare-ups, allowing for more informed choices regarding food intake during the warmer months.

Lastly, mental health can be particularly impacted in summer for those with eczema. The desire to enjoy outdoor activities while dealing with visible skin issues can lead to feelings of self-consciousness and anxiety. It is important for patients to prioritize mental well-being by engaging in activities that promote relaxation and self-care. Support groups or counseling can also provide valuable resources for managing the emotional aspects of living with eczema, ensuring that individuals feel supported and empowered throughout the summer season.

Adapting to Seasonal Changes

Adapting to seasonal changes is essential for managing eczema, as fluctuations in temperature, humidity, and environmental factors can significantly impact skin health. During colder months, the air tends to be drier, which can lead to increased skin dehydration. This dryness can exacerbate eczema symptoms, resulting in flare-ups characterized by itching, redness, and inflammation. It is crucial for patients to take proactive measures to maintain skin hydration, such as using a thick moisturizer regularly and employing a humidifier to add moisture to the indoor air.

In contrast, warmer months can introduce other challenges for individuals with eczema. Heat and sweat can trigger itching and discomfort, leading to scratching that worsens the condition. Patients should consider wearing lightweight, breathable fabrics and avoiding excessive sun exposure, which can irritate sensitive skin. Regular bathing with gentle, fragrance-free cleansers can help remove sweat and allergens while keeping the skin barrier intact. Incorporating an appropriate sunscreen is also vital to protect the skin from UV damage, which can lead to further complications.

Seasonal allergies can also play a significant role in eczema management. Pollen, mold, and other allergens can trigger inflammatory responses in the skin, leading to flare-ups. Patients should be aware of their local pollen counts and try to limit outdoor activities during peak seasons. Keeping windows closed, using air purifiers, and regularly cleaning indoor surfaces can help reduce allergen exposure. Identifying personal triggers is crucial in developing an effective management plan, as this knowledge empowers patients to minimize their risk of flare-ups during allergy season.

Dietary influences can also shift with the seasons, impacting eczema symptoms. Fresh fruits and vegetables become more available in warmer months, offering a variety of nutrients that can support skin health. Incorporating anti-inflammatory foods, such as fatty fish rich in omega-3s, can help reduce the severity of eczema symptoms. Conversely, during colder months, comfort foods may dominate diets, which can sometimes include ingredients known to trigger eczema. Patients should remain mindful of their dietary choices and consider keeping a food diary to identify any correlations between specific foods and their skin's condition.

Mental health is another critical aspect of adapting to seasonal changes in eczema management. The emotional toll of eczema can be heightened during specific seasons, especially when flare-ups coincide with holidays or social events. Patients should seek support from healthcare providers, join support groups, or engage in mindfulness practices to cope with the psychological impact of their condition. Understanding the interplay between seasonal changes, eczema symptoms, and mental health can help patients develop a more comprehensive approach to their overall well-being. This holistic perspective is vital for fostering resilience and maintaining a positive outlook while managing eczema throughout the year.

Chapter 10: Eczema-Related Allergies

Identifying Allergens

Identifying allergens is a crucial step in managing eczema symptoms effectively. Allergens are substances that can provoke an immune response, leading to inflammation and irritation of the skin. For individuals with eczema, understanding what triggers flare-ups can significantly improve their quality of life. Common allergens include pollen, pet dander, dust mites, mold, and certain foods. Patients should consider keeping a detailed diary to track their symptoms in relation to exposure to these potential allergens. This proactive approach can help identify patterns and pinpoint specific allergens that exacerbate their condition.

In infants and children, the identification of allergens is particularly important. Young skin is more sensitive and can react more severely to irritants and allergens. Parents should be vigilant about monitoring their child's environment and dietary intake. Introducing new foods gradually while observing for any adverse reactions can be beneficial. Discussing concerns with a pediatrician or an allergist can provide tailored advice and possibly lead to allergy testing, which can help in identifying specific triggers and guiding dietary adjustments.

Dietary influences play a significant role in eczema management. Certain foods, such as dairy, eggs, peanuts, and soy, are known to be common allergens that may worsen symptoms. It is essential for patients, especially those with eczema, to be cautious about their diet. An elimination diet, under the guidance of a healthcare professional, can assist in determining which foods may be contributing to flare-ups. After identifying problematic foods, patients can work on reintroducing them carefully, monitoring their skin's reaction to each.

Natural remedies can also aid in managing eczema symptoms related to allergens. Many patients find relief through the use of natural moisturizers and soothing agents, such as aloe vera or coconut oil, which can help calm irritated skin. Additionally, herbal treatments may provide anti-inflammatory benefits. However, it is imperative to ensure that these natural products do not contain allergens themselves. Conducting patch tests before widespread application can help determine skin sensitivity to new products.

Understanding the relationship between eczema and mental health is another essential aspect of identifying allergens and managing symptoms. The stress and anxiety associated with eczema flare-ups can create a vicious cycle, exacerbating symptoms. Patients should be encouraged to practice stress-reducing techniques, such as mindfulness or yoga, in conjunction with identifying and avoiding allergens. A holistic approach, addressing both physical and mental health, can lead to more comprehensive and effective management of eczema, ultimately improving overall well-being.

Skin Testing and Diagnosis

Skin testing plays a crucial role in diagnosing eczema and understanding its underlying causes. When patients present with symptoms such as dry, itchy, and inflamed skin, healthcare providers often recommend a series of skin tests to identify specific allergens or irritants that may be exacerbating the condition. These tests can include patch testing, prick testing, and intradermal testing, each designed to provoke a reaction that helps determine the source of the patient's discomfort. Understanding the results of these tests is essential for patients, as they can lead to more effective management strategies tailored to individual needs.

In infants and children, the diagnostic process may differ slightly due to their developing immune systems and skin barriers. Pediatric dermatologists are often tasked with distinguishing between eczema and other skin conditions that may present similarly, such as contact dermatitis or psoriasis. Skin testing in young patients typically involves careful consideration of their age and the safety of testing methods. Parents should be informed about the implications of test results and how they can influence dietary adjustments, skincare routines, and the overall management of eczema in their children.

Dietary influences on eczema are frequently a topic of discussion during the diagnostic phase. Some patients may experience flare-ups in response to specific foods, such as dairy, eggs, or nuts. An elimination diet, guided by a healthcare professional, can help identify potential food triggers. Skin testing can also be employed in conjunction with dietary assessments to pinpoint allergens that may not be immediately evident. Patients need to maintain open communication with their healthcare providers about their dietary habits and any observed correlations between food intake and eczema flare-ups.

Natural remedies are often considered by patients seeking alternative approaches to managing their eczema. During the diagnosis phase, it's important for patients to discuss any natural treatments they are using or considering, as some may interfere with conventional treatments or exacerbate symptoms. Healthcare providers can offer valuable insights into safe and effective natural remedies while ensuring that they do not compromise the overall management plan. Understanding the role of natural remedies within the context of a comprehensive treatment strategy can empower patients to make informed choices.

Lastly, the emotional impact of eczema cannot be overlooked during the diagnostic process. Patients may experience anxiety, frustration, or low self-esteem due to the visible nature of their symptoms. Healthcare providers should be attentive to the mental health aspects associated with eczema and may recommend counseling or support groups as part of the overall treatment plan. By addressing both the physical and emotional components of eczema, patients can work towards a holistic approach that not only targets symptoms but also supports their mental well-being.

Managing Allergies

Allergies play a significant role in the management of eczema, as they can exacerbate symptoms and lead to increased discomfort for individuals. Understanding the relationship between allergies and eczema is crucial for patients seeking to manage their condition effectively. Allergic reactions can trigger inflammation in the skin, causing flare-ups that may lead to itching, redness, and irritation. Identifying specific allergens—such as certain foods, pollen, pet dander, or dust mites—can help patients take proactive steps to minimize exposure and reduce the frequency and severity of eczema flare-ups.

For infants and children, the management of allergies is especially important, as their skin can be more sensitive and reactive. Parents should observe their child's reactions to various environmental factors and foods. Introducing new foods gradually, while monitoring for any adverse reactions, can help identify potential dietary influences that may worsen eczema. Additionally, maintaining a clean environment by reducing dust and allergens can create a more comfortable space for children with eczema, ultimately supporting their overall health and well-being.

Natural remedies can also aid in managing allergies related to eczema. Some patients find relief through herbal treatments, such as chamomile or calendula, which are known for their soothing properties. Other natural approaches include using essential oils or probiotics, which may help support the immune system and reduce allergic responses. It is essential for patients to consult healthcare professionals before incorporating any natural remedies into their routine to ensure safety and efficacy, particularly when treating young children or infants.

Mental health is another vital aspect of managing eczema and related allergies. The stress and discomfort caused by eczema can lead to anxiety or depression, compounding the difficulties associated with allergic reactions. Patients should prioritize self-care and consider seeking therapy or support groups to cope with the psychological impacts of their condition. Mindfulness practices, such as meditation or yoga, may help reduce stress levels and improve overall resilience against eczema flare-ups triggered by allergies.

Lastly, understanding seasonal changes is crucial for managing eczema and associated allergies. For many patients, certain seasons bring increased exposure to allergens, such as pollen in the spring or mold in the fall. Keeping track of the seasons and adjusting skincare routines and allergy management strategies accordingly can help minimize flare-ups. Regular consultations with healthcare providers can assist patients in developing a personalized management plan that addresses both eczema and allergies, ensuring a holistic approach to their skin health.

Chapter 11: Eczema Treatments and Medications

Over-the-Counter Options

Over-the-counter (OTC) options for managing eczema provide patients with accessible solutions that can help alleviate symptoms and improve skin condition. These products are available without a prescription and can be found in pharmacies, supermarkets, and online. Common OTC options include moisturizers, corticosteroid creams, antihistamines, and barrier repair creams. It is crucial for patients, particularly parents of infants and children with eczema, to understand which products may be most effective and how to use them safely.

Moisturizers are fundamental in an eczema management routine. A thick, emollient cream or ointment can help restore the skin barrier, reducing dryness and preventing flare-ups. Patients should look for products that are free of fragrance and irritants, as these can exacerbate symptoms. For infants and children, choosing pediatrician-recommended moisturizers can provide added peace of mind. Regular application of moisturizers, especially after bathing, can lock in moisture and help soothe inflamed skin.

Corticosteroid creams are another common OTC treatment for eczema flare-ups. These medications reduce inflammation and itching, offering quick relief during acute episodes. However, they should be used with care, particularly in children and those with sensitive skin. Patients should follow the instructions on the packaging regarding frequency and duration of use to avoid potential side effects, such as skin thinning or tolerance build-up. For mild cases, low-potency corticosteroids are often sufficient, while more severe cases may require higher-potency options.

Antihistamines can also be beneficial for managing eczema symptoms, especially when itching disrupts sleep. These medications can help reduce the urge to scratch, which is vital in preventing further irritation and secondary infections. Patients should opt for non-drowsy formulations during the day and consider sedating options at night to facilitate better sleep. It is essential to consult with a healthcare provider before starting any antihistamine to ensure it is appropriate for individual circumstances, particularly in young children.

Barrier repair creams are a newer category of OTC products designed to restore the skin's natural barrier function. These formulations often contain ingredients like ceramides and fatty acids that closely mimic the skin's own lipids. Regular use can help fortify the skin against irritants and allergens, which is particularly beneficial for patients with eczema triggered by environmental factors. When selecting a barrier repair cream, patients should look for those that are clinically tested for eczema and free from potential irritants. Integrating these OTC options into a comprehensive skincare routine can significantly improve overall skin health and enhance the quality of life for those affected by eczema.

Prescription Treatments

Prescription treatments for eczema are often necessary for patients who find that over-the-counter options do not provide sufficient relief from symptoms. These treatments are typically more potent and specifically formulated to target the inflammation, itchiness, and skin barrier dysfunction associated with eczema. Healthcare providers may recommend a range of topical and systemic medications based on the severity of the condition, the patient's age, and individual responses to previous treatments. Understanding these options can empower patients to engage in informed discussions with their healthcare providers about their treatment plans.

Topical corticosteroids are among the most commonly prescribed medications for eczema. They work by reducing inflammation and alleviating itching, making them effective in managing flare-ups. The strength of the corticosteroid prescribed can vary, with mild options suitable for delicate skin in infants and children, while stronger formulations may be necessary for adult patients with more severe symptoms. It is essential to follow the prescribed regimen closely, as overuse can lead to side effects such as skin thinning, particularly in sensitive areas.

In cases where topical treatments are insufficient, healthcare providers may consider immunomodulators. These medications, such as tacrolimus and pimecrolimus, help modulate the immune response in the skin, reducing inflammation without the side effects often associated with long-term use of corticosteroids. Immunomodulators can be particularly beneficial for sensitive areas like the face and eyelids, where corticosteroids may not be advisable. Patients must be educated about the proper application and potential side effects, including a burning sensation upon initial use.

For patients with moderate to severe eczema who do not respond to topical medications, systemic treatments may be necessary. These treatments include oral corticosteroids, cyclosporine, and newer biologic therapies like dupilumab. Biologics target specific pathways in the immune system, offering a more tailored approach to managing eczema. While these medications can be highly effective, they may come with significant costs and potential side effects, requiring careful monitoring by healthcare providers.

In addition to pharmacological treatments, it is vital for patients to integrate a comprehensive skincare routine as part of their management strategy. Prescription treatments should be complemented with regular moisturizing practices and avoidance of known triggers, such as harsh soaps and environmental irritants. Patients should also be aware of the impact of dietary influences on eczema and consider discussing dietary changes with their healthcare provider. By combining prescription treatments with lifestyle modifications, patients can achieve better control over their eczema symptoms and improve their overall quality of life.

Emerging Therapies

Emerging therapies for eczema represent a significant advancement in our understanding and management of this complex condition. As researchers continue to explore the underlying mechanisms of eczema, new treatment options are being developed that aim to address both the symptoms and the root causes of the disease. These therapies range from biologics, which target specific pathways involved in inflammation, to innovative topical treatments that offer enhanced efficacy and reduced side effects. For patients, staying informed about these emerging therapies can provide hope and new avenues for relief from eczema symptoms.

Biologics have gained attention as a revolutionary approach to eczema treatment, particularly for moderate to severe cases that do not respond to traditional therapies. These drugs work by inhibiting specific proteins involved in the inflammatory response, such as interleukin-4 and interleukin-13. By targeting these pathways, biologics can significantly reduce inflammation and improve skin barrier function. Patients considering biologics should discuss with their healthcare provider the potential benefits and risks, as well as the possibility of incorporating this treatment into their overall eczema management plan.

In addition to biologics, topical therapies are evolving with the introduction of new formulations and active ingredients. Products that incorporate newer agents like crisaborole or roflumilast offer alternatives to traditional corticosteroids, which can sometimes lead to skin thinning or other side effects with long-term use. Patients may find that these newer options provide effective symptom relief with a more favorable safety profile. It is essential to work closely with a dermatologist to identify the most suitable topical treatment based on individual symptoms and skin type.

Dietary influences on eczema are also an area of ongoing research. While food allergens can trigger flare-ups in some individuals, other dietary components may have protective effects. New studies are investigating the role of anti-inflammatory diets rich in omega-3 fatty acids, antioxidants, and probiotics in managing eczema symptoms. Patients are encouraged to consider dietary modifications under the guidance of a healthcare professional, as personalized nutrition approaches could complement their existing treatment regimen and improve their overall skin health.

Finally, the intersection of mental health and eczema is increasingly recognized, with emerging therapies focusing on the psychological aspects of chronic skin conditions. Cognitive-behavioral therapy (CBT) and mindfulness-based interventions have shown promise in helping patients manage the emotional burden of eczema. These therapies can equip patients with coping strategies, reduce anxiety related to flare-ups, and improve their overall quality of life. As eczema management evolves, it is crucial for patients to consider a holistic approach that encompasses both physical and mental health, ultimately leading to more comprehensive and effective care.

www.ingramcontent.com/pod-product-compliance
Lightning Source LLC
Chambersburg PA
CBHW051708250726
48653CB00007B/2914